Managing the Maze

A Handbook for Resident and Fellowship Physicians Navigating Decision Points Post-Training

Edward R. Sweetser, MD

AAPL

978-1-960762-45-0 print
978-1-960762-46-7 eBook

Published by **American Association for Physician Leadership, Inc.**
PO Box 96503 | BMB 97493 | Washington, DC 20090-6503

Website: www.physicianleaders.org

13 8 7 6 5 4 3 2 1

Copyedited, typeset, indexed, and printed in the United States of America

PUBLISHER
Nancy Collins

PRODUCTION MANAGER
Jennifer Weiss

DESIGN & LAYOUT
Carter Publishing Studio

COPYEDITOR
Patricia George

DEDICATION

I would like to thank my family for their encouragement in writing this book. My wife, Suzanne, has been especially helpful to me by giving me advice on the topics and editing what I've written. I would also like to thank my daughter Ashleigh and my two sons, Ted and Patrick, for their support during the writing process.

I would also like to thank all the residents I've worked with over the years and with whom I discussed many of the topics of this book. They reported to me that they have received no formal training in these areas and strongly encouraged me to write a book with guidance and advice for residents and fellows who are finishing their training and going into medical practice.

It is my hope that this book will assist these medical professionals in finding the path that leads to a long and productive medical career and a fulfilling life, both professionally and personally.

TABLE OF CONTENTS

ABOUT THE AUTHOR

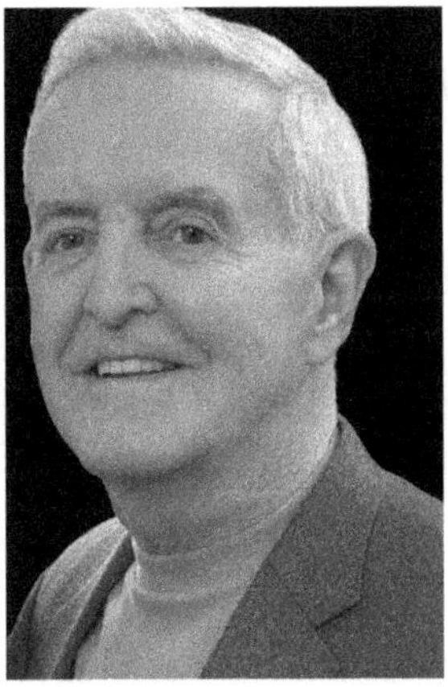

Edward R. Sweetser, MD, graduated from Georgetown University School of Medicine in Washington, DC, in 1970. He completed an Orthopedic Surgery Residency in 1975 at Georgetown University Hospital. From there he spent two years as an orthopedic surgeon in the United States Air Force in South Florida.

After discharge from the Air Force, he became employed by the Lovelace Clinic, a multi-specialty group practice and Medical Center in Albuquerque, New Mexico, as an orthopedic surgeon. He also was on the clinical faculty at the University of New Mexico Department of Orthopedic Surgery. While there, he published several articles in medical journals and presented at national orthopedic meetings. He also was the team physician for the Winter World University Games in Czeckoslovakia, 1987. He spent 15 years practicing and working with Residents in orthopedic surgery. During his last four-year tenure at Lovelace, he served as chief medical officer and obtained a Master's Degree in Health Services Administration.

In 1990, he joined a friend in private practice in Las Cruces, New Mexico, eventually growing the group to four surgeons. While there he had some contact with Family Practice Residents.

In 2002, he joined the medical staff of a new hospital in town, Mountain View Regional Medical Center, owned and built by Triad

Hospitals, later to be purchased by Community Health Systems (CHS). For five years he was still in private practice but in 2007 he decided to sell his practice assets and become employed by MountainView and CHS. During his years in practice at Mountain View he interacted with and taught Orthopedic Residents and served on the hospital's Medical Executive Committee.

He retired from clinical practice at Mountain View in 2020 and continued working as the chief medical officer for three years, fully retiring at the end of 2023. For the past 12 years, and continuing, he has served as a member of the Board of Trustees at Mountain View Regional Medical Center.

He has been happily married for 35 years to Suzanne Quillen, a nurse practitioner, who has been a hospital administrator for several years and is now vice president of innovation and CEO Training for a national Rehabilitation and Long-Term Acute Care Hospital System with 39 facilities in the United States. Together they share four children and four grandchildren.

PROLOGUE

When I finished my orthopedic surgery residency at Georgetown University Hospital in Washington, DC, I had no idea what kind of practice I wanted to pursue and had received no instruction about how to go about making any plans. My only experiences during medical school and residency were with faculty and private orthopedic practitioners.

I had some time to think about this decision, since I owed the U.S. Air Force two years. I was stationed at Homestead AFB, south of Miami and just north of the Florida Keys. The best part about the medical assignment was that the hospital and the clinics were in the same building.

We had clinics in multiple specialties and an active emergency room that cared for active-duty military members as well as retired veterans and their families. It was basically a group practice, and I found it very appealing to work with other physicians who saw each other on rounds, at lunch, and other times during the day, and with readily available consultations if needed.

Due to this experience, I sought group practice opportunities as I transitioned out of the military. I found a listing for the Lovelace Clinic in Albuquerque, New Mexico. It was a private clinic run by the Lovelace Medical Foundation with no other outside influences. We had more than 100 doctors and grew to almost 200 during my tenure.

Almost all specialties were represented. Our clinics and the hospital were in one location, and I found this to be a highly effective way to practice medicine. I was also on the orthopedic faculty at the University of New Mexico and worked daily with orthopedic residents.

After about 10 years, the Lovelace organization was partially taken over by HCA and an insurance company. In my opinion, the entire organization suffered. Much more attention was paid to profits rather than quality healthcare.

As the organization was changing in a way that I did not find satisfactory, I considered other practice options and looked in my specialty journal for alternative opportunities. I contacted an orthopedic surgeon I knew in Las Cruces, New Mexico, who was in a general orthopedic private practice. With the help of the local hospital providing an income guarantee, I joined my fellow orthopedist, who was working in a small building that he owned.

After a few years, we decided to move to a larger location. We found a vacant building that we believed had the potential to become a spacious office. We purchased the building and renovated it to meet our needs.

Being in private practice was quite different from the group practice I had been in. My partner and I developed a busy practice that required each of us to be on call one or two nights per week. We were responsible for hiring and managing staff, as well as billing and collecting.

We found this responsibility for finances to be extremely difficult and time-consuming. We typically collected 60% to 70% of what we billed. After a while, we found an outside billing agency that was able to increase our collections to more than 80% with a modest fee attached.

After we'd been practicing for about 10 years at this location, an outstanding and physician-friendly hospital group came to town with plans to build a new hospital. Another separate organization was planning to build a medical office building immediately adjacent to the new hospital.

We were offered what I considered a good financial deal to relocate from our building into the new building but maintain our own private practice. We worked with an architect provided by the building owners to determine the size and design of the new office.

With the final design in hand, my two partners decided that they would not accompany me to the new location.

From my perspective, this was a mistake since our current office was 20 minutes away from each of the two hospitals in town, and responding to emergency calls was very time-consuming and disruptive to the patients who were waiting to see us. I thought that being adjacent to the new hospital, which we could walk to easily and quickly, was much more efficient. So, with much trepidation, I went ahead with this project on my own.

The new hospital helped me recruit three new practitioners over the next two years, and I was able to find what I thought was a good office manager. Little did I know that the manager was skimming income collected in the office. The situation became complicated when three of the doctors decided to leave to establish their own orthopedic group in town. This was a very difficult time for me.

I was fortunate that the CEO of the hospital, now owned by a different for-profit hospital system, came forward and offered to purchase my equipment and accounts receivable and to hire me in an employed position. I would start receiving a salary and benefits after I signed the contract. This was an enormous relief for me in many ways.

I've been employed by the hospital for 15 years and have found this to be a much more satisfactory situation for me than private practice. The hospital assigned a new office manager to our office, who was knowledgeable and experienced, and the group hired some new staff and a few of the old staff. The hospital did all of the billing and collecting.

I had a basic income guarantee, along with productivity incentives and insurance benefits and coverage built into the contract. The contract was extensive, and even after more than 20 years in practice, I was a neophyte in the world of contracts. After personal consideration, I signed it. (We will discuss contracting in this book.)

I've spoken with the approximately 35 medical residents at my current hospital about their plans for after residency. We discussed what kind of practice they're going to look for, where they're going to live, and some of the ins and outs of employed and private practices. They have all shared that they received no formal training or education about the situations that they're going to face as they leave the residency program. I wrote this book to help young physicians master the maze of post-residency decision-making. I also address some of the areas new physicians will encounter, including licensing and hospital privileging, contracting, the malpractice insurance landscape, and emerging trends in the medical field. I hope the book will help doctors entering their post-residency years better evaluate new practice opportunities and compare one practice with another.

INTRODUCTION

Residency/Fellowship Is Coming to an End — What's Next?

Approximately 25,000–30,000 residents and 5,000–10,000 fellows complete their training each year and begin the next phase of their medical careers, according to the American Association of Medical Colleges (aamc.org). Many are unprepared to navigate the myriad choices that confront them. If you are within a year of completing your residency or fellowship, the end is in sight! You are probably thinking about what kind of practice you want and where you want to practice. Perhaps you're wondering how to find the right practice setting.

It is never too early to start thinking about these issues, as they can be time-consuming and include multiple decision points. Even after making the final decision, you must complete several steps before starting your new job.

There are substantially more options and considerations today than when I began this journey many years ago. The concept of hospitalists and intensivists had yet to be realized. Working for corporate America was not that common, and now, for-profit organizations, hospital corporations, and private equity-owned organizations have a stronghold on the purse strings of many hospitals and physician practices across the country.

When I embarked on my search, I knew little about things like contracts, paid time-off, retirement plans, benefits, and malpractice insurance. But those are critical considerations as you enter practice or move onto new venues over the years.

Unfortunately, most residents receive no formal instruction about the business considerations of going into practice and feel unprepared to address these issues.

I hope that this handbook will help you make choices that will result in a long and fulfilling career of taking care of our most precious resources: people.

CHAPTER 1

Considerations for Practice Opportunities

Lifestyle and personal time are, for the majority of residents, the most important considerations in choosing a job opportunity. A good financial package and geographic location are also important.

There are myriad practice opportunities, each with its own pros and cons. In this chapter, we will cover some of the more common practice situations available, each offering something distinct.

In the past, most physicians were recruited by either a hospital system or a private practice. Now the market has changed, and physicians are also being recruited by insurance companies, private equity groups, urgent care centers, retail clinics, federally qualified health centers, and telemedicine groups — all competing for the same pool of candidates.

The following are some of the more common practice opportunities available for physicians in the United States.

Entering Private Practice

Several years ago, most physicians aspired to private practice. Often, the young physician joined a physician or group that was already in private practice. Today, few graduating residents consider private practice, according to Becker's Physician Leadership.

Starting a new practice can be daunting, especially with the financial considerations. You must locate office space to buy or rent, outfit it with appropriate furniture and equipment, find staff, and pay them from day one. Obtaining malpractice insurance and defending against malpractice suits are critical and expensive aspects of owning a practice, especially in certain specialties, and the whole gamut of billing and collecting is complicated and can be frustrating.

Due to these intricacies, many physicians have gravitated away from private practice into an employed situation where all these considerations are covered by the employer. Today, it is estimated that 70% or more of physicians are employed in some capacity. As an employed physician, however, you do lose much of the autonomy and flexibility of a private practice.

For those who might want to consider establishing a private practice, the American Medical Association has excellent advice on its website in an article entitled "Starting Your Private Practice: An Entrepreneurial Guide to the Basics," by Daniel Choi, MD (https://www.ama-assn.org/practice-management/private-practices/starting-your-private-practice-entrepreneurial-guide-basics). Practice opportunities are available at JAMACareerCenter.com.

Establishing a Concierge Practice

Some private practice physicians have transformed their practice into a concierge model. In this model, a patient pays an annual fee to their primary care physician in exchange for enhanced access. The annual fee can range from a couple of thousand dollars to several thousand.

The physician agrees to be available to the patient beyond what would be the norm for a regular practice, such as same-day appointments, extended time per appointment, or 24/7 access to the physician. Many of these physicians also attend to patients who need to be admitted to the hospital.

The physician does not bill the patient for services, as the membership fee covers them. However, patients may be billed for lab work or specialist referrals. Some physicians have found this to be an easier and more effective way to remain in a private setting and avoid the administrative hassles of billing and collecting.

Joining a Specialty Group in Private Practice

Some physicians join an already-existing group in private specialty practice. They typically join as employees, under contract, with the possibility of becoming a partner over time.

The advantage of this type of practice is that it is already operational, with equipment, staff, and billing processes in place. Consequently, there is minimal upfront expense for the new physician. However, before embarking on such a practice, it is recommended that you evaluate several aspects of the practice, including:

- Finances and business practices.
- Market and competition.
- Group strategic direction.
- The path to becoming a partner, including associated time and costs.
- Other items, such as malpractice suits, planned upgrades, etc.

All these considerations should be to your liking before you agree to become a part of this type of practice.

Joining an Employed Group Practice

This type of practice is often organized by a hospital, a group of hospitals, or a for-profit organization, and is frequently associated with one or more medical office buildings. In most of these situations, the specialties are already in place and run by the organization's administration.

These practice models have become attractive to young physicians coming out of training and are worth serious consideration. They almost always require signing a contract that includes a variety of provisions presented as non-negotiable, but this is not always the case. In most of these situations, it will be necessary to have hospital privileges, which involves credentialing and privileging, which we will cover later.

These positions are appealing because you can walk right in and start practicing on day one with no upfront expenses and receive the agreed-upon compensation, often with no productivity metrics for the first year.

Joining a Major Organization

Seeking a position in a major organization, such as the Mayo Clinic, is a more competitive undertaking than being employed by a hospital. These organizations frequently seek out physicians who have established a reputation for reporting their research in scientific papers. Unless you have trained in one of these organizations, it is difficult to obtain a position directly out of residency or fellowship. See Appendix D for a list of major physician employers.

Working for an Academic Medical Center

Academic medical centers frequently recruit their own residents when there is a practice vacancy; however, these organizations may be seeking physicians who have established themselves in a university practice elsewhere and have written scientific research papers that have been published.

In addition to patient care and teaching, these positions also require physicians to take part in scholarly activity, which includes conducting research, writing papers for publication, and presenting at medical meetings. Most of these centers require employees to sign a contract before joining the group.

In some situations, especially those connected with the state, you immediately become a member of the state-run retirement plan. However, your employer will not be paying into Social Security for you while you work at the institution. In addition, if you leave this type of practice before you are eligible for the pension, you will need to pay into Social Security for 10 years to be able to qualify for these benefits.

Working for the Veterans Health Administration

The VHA provides care at 1,321 healthcare facilities, including 172 medical centers and 1,138 outpatient sites serving 9 million enrolled veterans each year. Many of the VA hospitals in the country are affiliated with major university medical centers. As such, they frequently recruit physicians from the resident training programs.

Some of the more desirable aspects of working for the VA system, as of this writing, are that you are eligible for generous federal retirement benefits, good insurance coverage, relatively stable employment with a competitive salary, regular pay increases, as well as 26 days of paid annual leave and paid parental leave.

The VA system also offers a contract buy-out program that allows the VA to recruit physicians and buy out their contractual obligation with their current employer in exchange for four years of service at one of the rural VA medical centers or affiliated community-based outpatient clinics.

Working in the Military

You may have received financial support from a branch of the military during medical school that requires active-duty time post-residency or fellowship. The military can assign you wherever they believe there is a need in the United States and around the world.

One of the enticing aspects of this job opportunity is the fact that after 20 years of service, you can retire with a reasonable pension and there is still an opportunity for practicing in an alternate setting before your final retirement.

Working in Nursing Homes or Prisons

These opportunities can be limited and, to a certain extent, confining and potentially not as rewarding, from a physician's perspective.

Taking Locum Positions

Locum tenens positions are usually time-limited at a specific location but frequently pay reasonably well. In some cases, you may only work a week or two a month. These positions usually provide a housing allowance and expenses but may not be in what you consider a desirable location.

Because the position is temporary, you may need to move from one location to another with some frequency and be away from your family for an extended period of time. On the other hand, you may find the practice opportunity appealing and might even consider settling permanently in a location after your *locums* work. *Locum* agencies can help you find a desirable practice location and also assist you with licensure in the states in which you work. See Appendix B for a list of *locum* agencies.

Practicing Telemedicine

You can become a full-time employed telemedicine physician in a variety of organizations, which typically requires being licensed in more than one state so you can treat patients in several locations.

Some physicians use telemedicine as a part of their practice to facilitate healthcare for patients who live a significant distance from their practice location. This can be a complicated process for patients who are not well-versed in computer or smartphone technology.

One of the nice things about this type of practice is that you do not need an office or staff, and the billing and collection are done by the organizations that employ you. In some cases, you will need your own malpractice insurance if the telehealth company does not offer it. See Appendix J for a list of telemedicine companies.

CHAPTER 2

Determining the Right Practice Opportunity

Finding a practice opportunity can be a long and arduous process. Therefore, I strongly recommend that you start looking at least a year before you finish your residency. After you decide on a practice and location, you must obtain a license from the state and get credentialed by the organization, the hospital, and the insurance payers. These steps can take three or more months to complete, and you cannot start practicing until it's all taken care of, so begin as soon as possible.

A year or two before finishing your residency, you likely will receive inquiries or offers from recruiters about opportunities around the country. Some may be appealing and worthy of a response; most of them you will probably discard.

It is important to understand that the employer, not the physician, pays the physician recruiting firms. Due to the high costs involved, small groups and private practices often avoid working with recruiters, and those that do may offer a lower salary to offset the cost of using recruiters. Approximately 80% of physicians who don't use recruiters and search firms earn between $10,000 and $40,000 more than those who use a recruiter, according to Justin Nabity's 2024 article on Physicians Thrive (https://physiciansthrive.com/merritt-hawkins-review/).

Benefits of working with a physician recruiter include access to their extensive network and the recruiter's ability to speed up the hiring process. Some recruiting services can help you write your CV, assess a practice opportunity, and understand various practice settings. They can also provide helpful insights on how to interview and what questions to ask of your potential new employer.

Additionally, recruiters are well-versed in fair market value for physicians and their specialties in the region in which you might be interested. They can let you know if the compensation and benefits package of your potential employer is on par with your specialty and the location.

Physician recruiters also may help you obtain a higher signing bonus, a higher relocation fee, and a higher CME allowance. They can be invaluable in helping you navigate the contract process.

If the recruitment company does not offer counsel regarding contracts, it may be wise to work with a contract review specialist before signing any documents. Some large law firms have specialists in physician contract terms and negotiations, but there is a cost associated with their services.

Looking Beyond Recruiters

Other sources of job opportunities include:

Medical search firms. Many medical search firms may have job opportunities that are not posted publicly. Several of these firms are listed in Appendix A. The people you contact at these firms can give you information about the practice and, in some situations, can help you negotiate for pay and benefits. These negotiations can be daunting, and having help from experienced professionals can make the process easier and more worthwhile for you.

The internet. You'll have no problem locating specialty-specific medical jobs by searching the internet. Unfortunately, for most of these postings, the information listed is minimal. They might not include such basic information as the location and the general salary range. Responding to the post may connect you with a recruiter who can give you more specific information about the practice opportunity.

Publications. Specialty-specific journals often feature advertisements for open positions that provide details about the type of practice and its location, but typically require a personal contact at the organization to obtain additional information.

Conferences. Some of the larger medical specialty meetings provide booths for recruiters to interact with job seekers and discuss opportunities that may or may not be published elsewhere. Establishing a personal relationship with these recruiters can be advantageous as you pursue a practice opportunity.

Social media. Doximity is a medical social media site that often posts practice opportunities in specialties, giving you direct contact with the recruiter or with the organization.

***Locum tenens* companies.** Another option to consider, as described in the previous chapter, is *locum tenens* positions. Many facilities need temporary coverage in certain specialties. In some cases, it may be for a couple of weeks; sometimes the need is for a month or two. These positions generally pay well and include payment for travel, housing, and malpractice insurance coverage.

Locum tenens work gives you the opportunity to get a feel for the community, the facility, and the job opportunity at that facility. And it also gives the facility and the administrators an opportunity to see you in action and to develop a relationship that could lead to a permanent position for both of you. This can also be the ultimate site visit.

Some physicians use these temporary assignments to supplement their core income or pay down student debt. See Appendix B for a list of some of the larger *locums* firms.

Professional contacts. It is not unusual that residency and fellowship directors have personal contacts with outside organizations. If you ask them, they may be able to provide guidance on which positions might be available, as well as the contact information for the relevant locations if you are interested. These individuals can also help you prepare for recruiting visits and interviews.

As you begin your search, it is also worth reviewing Appendix C, which provides a list of best and worst states for physicians based on opportunity-competition and medical environment.

CHAPTER 3

Tips for Making Contact

When you've identified one or more opportunities that seem to be a good fit for you, it's time to take the next step. When responding to recruiting ads or inquiries, it's often beneficial to provide a cover letter that outlines your background, skills, and abilities, and an up-to-date CV with accomplishments that show you in a good light. This is not always required, but it is a way to distinguish yourself from other potential applicants who may not provide such additional information.

Responding to job postings by phone or email frequently puts you in contact with a national or local recruiter. Many larger organizations and hospitals have onsite recruiters whom you will contact directly when you respond to the posting. The recruiter can provide you with more detailed information about the posting.

If, after hearing about the location and the opportunity, you want to pursue the position, the recruiter may arrange for you to speak to the CEO of the organization or another member of the administrative staff. During these initial contacts, there is usually very little discussion about the specifics of a contractual relationship beyond a brief conversation about salary and benefits, including a sign-on bonus.

During the discussion, you are trying to get a feel for the practice and location, and they are assessing whether you would be a good fit for the organization. If they are interested in you, they typically will contact you within a couple of days and invite you for an onsite visit.

CHAPTER 4

Navigating the Site Visit and Following Up

Most recruiters advise residents who are beginning their first physician job search to start 18 months to two years before the completion of training. Start early, but be selective and only entertain interview invitations that genuinely interest you. Onsite interviews are time-consuming and can be taxing emotionally, so be intentional with your acceptances.

Site visits are perhaps the most important element of the recruitment process. If you are not offered a site visit, I recommend that you do not pursue the opportunity. You cannot get a good feeling for the organization, the medical staff, or the location without visiting the site. I encourage you to also request that your significant other be allowed to accompany you on the visit. I have witnessed many offers to interested physicians whose spouse or partner came for a look and was less than enthusiastic for whatever reason.

Once you begin your search, narrow down your top three opportunities and schedule those onsite visits within weeks of each other. Scheduling multiple site visits over several months can prove problematic for many reasons, but the main reason is that if this is a high-demand specialty, your top offer could be filled by the time you complete all your site visits and make a decision.

If you are sold on one offer, don't continue your search for the sake of more site visits. If you believe the position fits at least 80% of your practice criteria, accept the offer and cancel the remainder of your scheduled site visits.

Preparing for the Interview

The specifics of the site visit are typically handled by the recruiter or organization representative with whom you have had contact.

They will help you select a date and arrange your transportation and accommodations. Your contact will also arrange meetings between you and the CEO, practice administrator, and other administrative staff as applicable.

They will arrange for you to visit the practice location and, as appropriate, the hospital and its facilities, and will introduce you to the relevant administrators at these sites. They will also arrange for you to meet with physicians in your specialty as well as physicians from other specialties. If you are interviewing for a group practice, they will likely arrange for you to see some of the other facilities in and around the town.

Here are some additional recommendations for your visit:

- Prepare for your site visit by researching the practice, hospital, or clinic as well as the community.
- Arrive on time. If you can't determine from the itinerary where you should be at a particular time, ask in advance.
- Dress professionally and DO NOT WEAR SCRUBS!
- Ask questions that demonstrate you have done your research on the organization.
- Bring copies of your CV to distribute at meetings.
- Be prepared to sell yourself and your special skills and abilities.
- Be considerate of those you meet.
- Avoid discussing other opportunities you may be pursuing.

When meeting with the assigned personnel, especially the CEO, practice administrator, or lead physician, you must communicate effectively. Consider mirroring what they say by repeating it and agreeing with it, if indeed you do agree. Use open-ended questions to gather more information about issues. For example, you might ask. "What are the considerations for a salary increase?" rather than saying, "I would like an increase in my salary."

Here are some questions to ask:

- How many practitioners exist in my specialty?
- Is my specialty needed, and will I be expected to practice it in this group?

- What is the general pay scale for my specialty in this part of the country?
- What are my on-call requirements?
- If I am a proceduralist, will I have assigned times given to me?
- Is there more than one practice location that I'm required to use or cover?
- What are my benefits? And do I get them at the start of practice, especially time off?
- When will I hear if you are interested in me?

You should understand your call responsibilities in the hospital and/or office, the productivity expected of you, and the kind of computer systems you will be using if you choose to join the group. Get a feel for where the group is headed in the future and what your specific responsibilities will be.

It is also critical that you become familiar with the people with whom you will be working. This requires a give-and-take approach at group meetings. Ask who left the organization or practice recently and why. If appropriate, ask how and when you might have an opportunity to become a partner in the group.

While in town, you and your spouse or significant other should meet with a real estate agent for a tour of the community. Ask about housing costs and the standard of living. Discover what the community has to offer and what the schools' quality ratings are.

Letter of Intent

After the site visit, you'll probably meet with the CEO or other critical members of the facility or practice to discuss the outcome of the site visit from your perspective as well as from the perspective of the organization. If there is mutual agreement about bringing you into the organization, the organization will usually present you directly, or soon thereafter, with a letter of intent (LOI) that outlines in more detail some of the specifics of the offer, such as:

- A guaranteed salary for a specified period.
- Productivity expectations.
- Sign-on bonus.

- Debt payment offering.
- Relocation expenses and/or support.
- Malpractice coverage.

This is not the final contract. After you sign the letter of intent, it is usually followed shortly thereafter with an official contract. Ideally, this occurs at least six to nine months before your expected start date, allowing you to obtain a medical license in that state and secure your privileges at the hospital and with the insurers so that you can begin practicing on your official first day.

Note: After each step of this process, but especially after the onsite interview, it is essential to express your gratitude for their time and interest by sending a personalized email or handwritten note to those you met, thanking them individually.

CHAPTER 5

Evaluating the Employment Contract

After you send back the signed letter of intent, you will receive the employment contract. The contract is often presented as a take-it-or-leave-it, but this is not necessarily the case.

There may be opportunities for negotiation, especially if your specialty or subspecialty is in high demand. Most physicians feel uncomfortable about or are not prepared for negotiating with the practice administrator.

The American Medical Association offers information about physician employment contracts on its website. In addition, KevinMD.com offers guidance on contract negotiations and details of some common pitfalls, including:

- **Accepting the first offer:** Always negotiate for better terms.
- **Focusing solely on salary:** Consider the entire package, including benefits, working conditions, and exit provisions.
- **Failing to prepare:** Preparation is crucial for effective negotiation.
- **Letting emotions take over:** Keep your emotions in check and stay focused on your objectives.
- **Neglecting legal and professional advice:** Seek guidance from mentors or legal professionals.

It's also good to have a backup plan if you cannot negotiate the contract terms that are most important to you.

Some attorneys and organizations provide contract negotiation services for physicians. (See Appendix E for a list of law firms that help with physician contracting.) One of the benefits of using an experienced contract negotiator is that it takes the physician out of what may be an uncomfortable situation.

Generally, there is not much room for negotiation unless you are an attractive candidate due to your subspecialty or the organization's specific needs. In that case, they may be willing to negotiate with you about some of the specifics of the contract.

Negotiations aside, having an experienced lawyer or adviser review the contract can help you understand some of the contract's nuances that may be unfamiliar to you. As with contract negotiation services, there is a financial cost associated with working with consultants.

Basic Contract Terms

Start Date: The contract usually specifies a start date. If you have planned well, you will have plenty of time to obtain a state medical license, obtain hospital privileges and Medicare/insurance company approvals, and arrange for the move. The start date may be adjusted if you are unable to fulfill these requirements before the official start date in the contract.

Term Length: The term of the initial contract is usually designated in years, such as one or two years, before it terminates and is subject to renegotiation.

Board Certification Timeline: If you're finishing a residency or fellowship and have completed a certain amount of time in practice, you are qualified to take the board examination in your specialty. Board certification and time-limited board eligibility are required for licensing in some states and for continuing your privileges at a hospital. This may be specified in the contract.

Practice Location: This element is oftentimes specified in the contract and may involve one or more practice locations for your specialty. You should have been aware of and seen these practice locations during the initial site visit. Ensure the contract clearly outlines your responsibilities at each of these locations.

Duties: Your specific duties with the organization, such as a particular subspecialty, will usually be incorporated in the contract.

Call Coverage: The specifics of the practice and/or hospital call requirements are included in the contract, including the number of days of hospital call required. In some situations, even though your primary duties may be in your subspecialty, you may be required to take general specialty call for the hospital. Ensure you are aware of these requirements before signing the contract.

Restrictions on Outside Activities: Some contracts may include provisions that restrict you from certain activities, such as consulting, telemedicine, or other healthcare provider activities.

Residential Restrictions: Some contracts specify that you must live within a certain distance of the medical facility, especially if you are required to take call at the facility.

Contract Finances

Compensation: A specific salary will be identified for a particular duration. This number is usually obtained from a national database, often the Medical Group Management Association, and is based on specialty and location. Salaries may vary significantly depending on the location of the practice.

The contract may specify that the salary is based on the fair market value (FMV) of the specialty and the location. FMV is the salary and benefits that a physician can reasonably expect to be offered in a specific market and timeframe by specialty.

Although an employer may state that the salary is non-negotiable, it still may be negotiated based on your specific skills and the need for your services in that area. See Appendix F for salary ranges by specialty.

Most finishing residents and fellows would prefer to receive a set salary with production bonuses. This is a common method of compensation arrangements, although it is frequently overshadowed by the productivity-based payment methodology.

The initial contract often outlines what is expected in terms of productivity for a specific practice. This is usually based on the work relative value units (wRVUs) for a specific time frame. It may also be based on the number of patients to be seen for a given period, or for medical billings during a specific period.

During the first year or two, the physician's salary is usually fixed, but the salary for succeeding years is frequently based on one or more of these formulas. It is critical to understand what the current specialists are doing in terms of productivity and the relationship to salary before signing the contract. This will give you a better understanding of what to expect from your practice and your salary in future years.

Usually, a new salary is proposed at the end of the contract term, based on a productivity formula that is often specified elsewhere in the contract. This productivity formula may be based on RVUs, patient visits, or billings.

Typically, it takes at least a year to develop an active practice, but the total billings for the year are used to calculate the new salary, and often, the early billings are low. This can be detrimental in determining a new salary level. It would be wise to negotiate the new salary based on your productivity over the previous six months.

Claw Back Provisions: In some contracts, if your productivity does not meet expectations for a specified period, the organization may reduce your pay (claw back) during the upcoming month(s) to reflect this shortage in productivity expectations. This can be disconcerting, especially if you have taken approved time off (vacation) during that period.

Sign-on Bonus: The organization you're joining may give you a sign-on bonus in the initial contract. This may or may not be connected to other compensation, such as relocation expenses, debt payments, or CME expenses. Make sure you understand the specifics of this provision before you sign. Find out how long the sign-on bonus is active and if it needs to be repaid should you decide to leave.

Relocation Expenses: The contract will likely include a sum for relocating to the new location. This may or may not be tied to a total package of payments in the contract.

Student Loan Payment: Some contracts may include an offer to pay a certain amount of your debts related to schooling and moving expenses associated with the residency or fellowship programs. The total payment offered can be negotiated depending on your situation. For most physicians, this is an important consideration when making a decision about a position.

Note that for most of these reimbursements related to relocation expenses and student loans, if you decide to leave the organization before a specified period, you will be required to repay some or all the money that was given to you. It is important that you clearly understand this provision, as it may involve a substantial sum of money.

Board Certification and/or CME Expenses: Some organizations may compensate you for expenses related to board certification. In addition, most employed practices allocate a specific sum for CME expenses.

Employment Benefits

Usually, the specific benefits offered are detailed in separate benefit plan documents. These benefits are generally not negotiable and apply equally to all physicians within the organization. They include health insurance, disability insurance, and life insurance.

Retirement Plan: Most organizations offer a 401(k) or another similar plan that allows you to contribute up to a certain percentage of your salary. The organization may match a portion of your contribution. This plan is typically offered by a large nationwide organization, such as Fidelity, and allows you some control over the investment options.

Some state-run organizations, the Veterans Administration system, the military system, as well as the federal system, may have a pension plan that pays you a certain percentage of your final years' income for the rest of your life after you have reached a certain age and time with the organization. In these situations, no money is paid into Social Security. If you leave the organization before you are eligible for the pension, you will not qualify for Social Security benefits unless you start working for another organization where you and the new organization pay into Social Security for the specified time required (10 years) to be able to receive benefits.

Health Insurance: Most healthcare organizations offer health insurance that may include a dental plan and a vision plan. In some situations, if you receive your care at the organization and/or hospital, any expenses not covered by insurance may be waived.

Disability Insurance: Hopefully, you will not have to use this benefit, but you should consult with an experienced insurance adviser about this benefit soon after starting employment, as some employer-sponsored disability insurance plans do not pay adequately to match your annual salary and may be time-limited. They are also subject to change at the employer's discretion.

Consider obtaining your own disability insurance plan from a qualified broker to overcome some of these inadequacies. If you leave your new organization, especially if you do so at an older age and/or with some existing medical issues, it may be impossible to obtain this insurance, or it may be prohibitively expensive. For a young physician starting out, disability insurance is relatively inexpensive, and it is easy to increase the coverage as you age and your salary increases.

Family Leave Policy: A family leave policy is usually included in the overall benefit package per the federal Family and Medical Leave Act (FMLA). The FMLA provides eligible employees with up to 12 weeks of unpaid, job-protected leave per year for certain family and medical reasons. The policy will outline who qualifies for paid family leave, as well as how much time can be taken off and whether it's paid. FMLA typically covers maternity and paternity leave. The employer must maintain group health benefits during this leave time.

Vacation: The limitations for paid time off (PTO) are usually specified in the benefit plan. The number of hours may increase depending on how long you stay with the organization. Find out if you can carry over vacation time from year to year or if it is a "use it or lose it" situation. It's also good to know if you will be paid for unused vacation time if and when you leave the organization.

Note: If your salary is based on productivity, being away for an extended period of time can negatively impact your productivity and, in turn, your compensation when you return.

Malpractice Insurance Coverage: All employed physicians are covered by malpractice insurance. Some private practices leave this benefit up to each physician in the group. There are two types of malpractice insurance coverage: claims-made and occurrence-based.

Claims-made malpractice insurance covers you only if the policy is in effect at the time the malpractice claim is filed. If you let the policy lapse because you resigned or were terminated, you are not covered if a claim is filed. The only way you can be covered in this situation is if you purchase your own "malpractice tail coverage," which is quite expensive.

Occurrence-based malpractice insurance covers you for claims that are made for situations that occurred while the policy was in effect, even if you left the practice or retired.

Discuss with the risk manager any state-specific malpractice coverages. Also discuss the issue of punitive damages. If you lose a malpractice case, the plaintiff may pursue damages for the harm that resulted from your actions. These damages are not covered by malpractice insurance and must be paid out of your own personal proceeds. Find out how the organization covers this possible occurrence.

Contract Termination

Most contracts specify that either you or the organization can terminate the contract with or without cause if notification is made within a specific time period. Pay close attention to these termination clauses and understand your rights up front. Ideally, both parties should have a 90-day notification before the termination is final. This gives you time to find another practice to join and ensures your income during this time.

There are several other clauses to consider with regard to contract termination.

Restrictive Covenant: Many contracts state that if you leave or are terminated, you are restricted from practicing in the community or within a specified mileage of the facility. This is commonly called a noncompete clause. The idea is that your patients can't follow you to a new organization. This can create a significant financial burden for you.

The Federal Trade Commission recently finalized a rule banning most noncompete agreements, but the ruling has been challenged and is not currently resolved. Still, some states ban these covenants, so find out the status of this law in the state you will be practicing in.

Nonsolicitation and Nondisclosure Clauses: These clauses prohibit you from soliciting anybody on your staff and/or any current patients to join you in your new location. You may be prevented from having access to your patients' medical records unless specifically requested by the patients. Additionally, you agree to protect any confidential information shared with you by your employer.

Payback Clauses: As discussed earlier, if you leave the organization before a specified time, you may be required to repay some or all the money advanced to you for moving expenses, loan payments, bonuses, or other funds already paid to you.

Dispute Resolution

In many contracts, a method for dispute resolution is outlined, such as arbitration, mediation, and litigation.

The best way to avoid a dispute is to be familiar with every aspect of the contract — especially the salary and benefit package. I recommend consulting with an employment attorney before signing a contract.

Contract Errors to Avoid

In a November 6, 2024, *Medscape Medical News* article, Nicole Pajer discusses several errors physicians make when agreeing to an employment contract:

1. **Failing to Negotiate.** A potential employer needs you and wants you to be happy in the new organization, especially if

you have a needed subspecialty. So, talk up your strengths and don't be afraid to ask for what's not in the contract.

2. **Not Prioritizing Work-Life Balance.** Issues such as call schedules and vacation time can have a significant impact on your work-life balance and can lead to burnout. So don't hesitate to ask for more information about these issues and consider them carefully.
3. **Overlooking the Noncompete Clause.** This clause can seriously affect where you can live and work if you leave the organization for any reason. Consider asking for a limited mile radius from the facility, such as 5–7 miles, and consider telling the employer that if you leave, you will continue referring to the employed physicians and to the hospital and its diagnostic facilities.
4. **Breezing Past Malpractice Insurance.** In some situations, especially in a private group, malpractice insurance may be significantly higher for the new physicians. Check with your colleagues and see what they are paying, and then try to negotiate with the carrier for a better rate for yourself.
5. **Jumping Too Fast at a Signing Bonus.** Carefully evaluate the repayment obligations of any signing bonuses and ask that the bonus be prorated over a specified number of years so you are not stuck with a high bill if you decide to leave the group before the payout period is reached.
6. **Not Protecting Your Intellectual Property.** If you join an academic group where you will be doing research, there may not be any room to negotiate on this issue. But, if you join another type of organization, you should ensure that anything that you develop on your own that produces a financial reward will be yours alone.
7. **Underthinking Compensation Models.** A compensation model that emphasizes productivity units such as patients seen per day or surgeries performed, with no consideration for patient satisfaction or clinical outcomes, should be negotiated, as it can be stressful to meet these demands at all costs.

8. **Not Planning an Exit Strategy.** Evaluate the notice period for termination with or without cause. You will want a longer termination period if your employer terminates you, but a shorter period if you choose to leave for any reason.

Alert: If, after reviewing the contract in depth and attempting negotiation, you are not satisfied with the terms, be prepared to walk away and find another situation that better suits your needs.

CHAPTER 6

The Medical Licensing Process

All residents must hold a temporary or provisional license, also called a training license/certificate, to care for patients under faculty supervision in an accredited residency program until they are fully licensed. Some graduate medical education institutions and states may insist that a physician be fully licensed at a certain point in their training.

In the United States, medicine is a licensed profession and regulated by the individual states. One of the most important functions of the nation's state medical boards is issuing licenses to physicians. Through licensing, state medical boards ensure that all practicing physicians have appropriate education and training and that they abide by recognized standards of professional conduct while serving their patients.

While every physician must be licensed to practice medicine, board certification is voluntary. Some hospital bylaws require physicians to be board-certified or board-eligible to apply for and maintain clinical privileges. Medical licensure sets the minimum competency requirements to diagnose and treat patients and is not specialty-specific, whereas board certification demonstrates a physician's exceptional expertise in a particular specialty and/or subspecialty of medical practice.

Obtaining a Medical License

Obtaining a medical license can be a long and arduous process that varies from state to state. Contact the state licensing board to request a copy of its licensing requirements and inquire about the average time it takes to process applications. This will give you a better idea of a reasonable start date with your new employer and guide your relocation timeline. Providing the licensing board with a resume or Curriculum Vitae when you first make contact will allow the licensing board to evaluate potential problem areas early in the process.

Licensing boards can be complex, and their requirements can vary from state to state, depending on each jurisdiction's resources, regulations, and laws. The current licensure process requires physicians to complete individual applications for each state in which they seek to practice medicine in any form, including telemedicine. When applying for a license, you must submit all required documentation, including educational transcripts, exam scores, and residency verification. The following is a comprehensive list of general requirements:

General Requirements for a State Medical License

- Proof of medical school degree.
- Proof of successful passage of all three parts of the Medical Licensing Examination or the Comprehensive Osteopathic Medical Licensing Examination.
- At least one year of an ACGME residency program, or a foreign program approved by the state.
- Fingerprint cards.
- Driver's license.
- Notarized copy of birth certificate or current valid passport.
- Supporting documentation of legal name change.
- Copy of your specialty board certificate or proof of residency training.
- Proof of compliance with immigration laws if a non-citizen: naturalization papers, passport, J-1, or H-1 Visa.
- Passport-sized photo.
- Health status (physical and mental).
- Proof of malpractice insurance and the name of the company.
- CV or resume.
- Professional references (usually two or three) from physicians who have recent (within the past two or three years) direct personal knowledge of your character and competence to practice medicine.

- Verification of work experience for the preceding five years.
- Hospital privileges from all hospitals where you have worked.
- Other verified medical licenses.
- Disclosure of all actions that may be on your record: legal actions, behavior issues, disciplinary actions, malpractice actions, academic-related actions, and others, such as a criminal background check.

Note: Be forthcoming in explaining the circumstances of any action against you. In most cases, medical boards are understanding. Also, making a false statement on an application can be grounds for denial or future restriction.

During the application process, you may consider using Hospital Services Corporation credentials verification or the Federation Credentials Verification Service (FCVS), which verifies and stores your documents, making it easy to apply for licenses in several states.

FCVS (fsmb.org/fcvs) is a service of the Federation of State Medical Boards (FSMB) and provides a centralized, uniform process for state medical boards as well as private, governmental, and commercial entities to obtain a verified primary source record of a physician's core credentials. It establishes a permanent lifetime repository of primary source verified core credentials, including medical education, postgraduate training, examination history, board action history, board certification, and identity for physicians and physician assistants.

Currently, 97% of state boards accept or require applicants to use FCVS. This repository can be forwarded, at the applicant's request, to nearly any state medical board, hospital, healthcare facility, or other entity.

The Uniform Application (UA) makes the licensure application process easier by eliminating redundancy. When you complete the UA online, your application is securely stored and can be resubmitted to another state board using the UA without reentering the same information. You would only need to make updates as needed and ensure that you comply with any state medical board-specific requirements.

You would benefit from enrolling in FCVS to have your credentials verified and accessible when you're ready to apply for your first full and unrestricted license to practice medicine. You can learn more about this at the FCVS website.

Required Examinations

The United States Medical Licensing Examination (USMLE) provides state medical boards with a common evaluation system for licensure applicants. The exam is administered by the National Board of Medical Examiners (NBME) and sponsored by NBME and the Federation of State Medical Boards (FSMB). The USMLE consists of three separate exams, known as steps.

Step 1 assesses the basic sciences taught during the pre-clerkship curriculum. Step 1 is generally taken upon completing the pre-clerkship curriculum.

Step 2 assesses clinical knowledge and skills that can be applied to patient care under supervision. Step 2 is usually taken after concluding medical school clinical rotations.

Step 3 assesses in-depth clinical knowledge and decision-making to be able to care for patients independently. Step 3 is typically taken after the first year of residency.

You may be required to take and pass the Comprehensive Osteopathic Medical Licensing Examination. This is a three-level exam administered by the National Board of Osteopathic Medical Examiners (NBOME). All osteopathic medical students are required to pass COMLEX-USA level 1 and level 2 during medical school and level 3 during residency.

The licensure board will verify all information you submit to them. This primary source verification (PSV) for physicians is typically carried out by the Federation Credentials Verification Service (FCVS). Some states use the Hospital Services Corporation (HSC) Credentials Verification Organization. Residents are advised to follow up with the state medical boards and to respond to any requests for additional information in a timely fashion. This expedites the medical licensure process.

Foreign Medical Graduates

For foreign medical graduates to obtain a U.S. residency, they must have an MD degree or equivalent, have passed USMLE Step 1 and Step 2, have an Educational Commission for Foreign Medical Graduates (ECFMG) certification, and obtain a Visa, if indicated.

International medical graduates may need to obtain a status report of the certification and request certification of successful completion of the 5th pathway program, if applicable, directly from the school. They will also need to send examination scores from USMLE, Flex, National Board, and ECFMG certification to the state medical board. For applicants certified by ECFMG, an ECFMG certification status report is included in each profile forwarded to a state board. This report is required by all state boards, except Maryland, and is state-specific, proprietary, and valid for one year from issue date. A $66 fee is incurred for each state board designation.

Additional Considerations

License Renewal: The process of renewing a license varies from state to state, but typically requires at a minimum, proof of continuing medical education, passing of licensure exams, and submission of personal and professional documents. Renewal deadlines vary from 6 to 24 months from initial issuance, so it's essential to pay attention to expiration dates and follow all renewal processes.

Fast Track: The Interstate Medical Licensure Compact (IMLC) offers an expedited pathway to licensure for qualified physicians who wish to practice in multiple states. It is designed to facilitate telemedicine services and to increase access to care in areas with physician shortages. As of December 2025, 37 states, Guam, and the District of Columbia are participating members. To learn more, visit www.imlcc.org.

National Practitioner Data Bank: Many state medical boards require physicians to supply a National Practitioner Data Bank (NPDB) self-query report as part of the licensure process. Several state medical boards have designated FSMB as an authorized agent to request an NPDB report on their behalf, resulting in reduced time and costs. Each FCVS profile delivered to a participating board will include a unique one-time NPDB report.

Professional Licensure Groups: Residents may find it beneficial to hire a professional licensing service for their initial medical licensure application, thereby increasing their chances of approval and saving time and effort. These agencies offer accurate and timely processing and maintain contact with the board reviewer until your license is granted. This takes a lot of the pressure off you when you are trying to focus on your residency.

The licensing service also keeps your records stored and available if you apply to another state for a license or need to provide your credentials to another hospital, medical group, or agency. There are charges for these services, but it may be worth it to have this information readily available in an electronic format should you decide to apply for other state licenses.

After You Have Your License

After obtaining your medical license, you will need to register with the state board of pharmacy in order to write prescriptions for controlled substances. You will need to obtain your Controlled Substances Registration (CSR) and your DEA Certification from the Drug Enforcement Administration. These certifications are obtained online at state and federal sites, respectively.

For the DEA certification, you will need to complete a one-time eight-hour training course on the treatment and management of patients with opioid or other substance use disorders. While a DEA number is not technically required for prescribing non-controlled substances, practicing without one can cause a lot of problems.

Using DEA numbers gives pharmacies and insurance companies a simple, standardized method for identifying providers when processing claims for prescription medications. Most hospitals and healthcare organizations require both a CSR and a DEA number, with all classes listed on them to ensure that a provider does not prescribe a class of medication that is not listed on their CSR and DEA.

Additional resources can be found at the Accreditation Council for Graduate Medical Education website (www.acgme.org) and the Association of American Medical Colleges website (www.aamc.org).

CHAPTER 7

The Credentialing and Privileging Process

Credentialing and privileging are the next steps after you've received licensure. A medical license is issued by a state or federal agency and ensures the physician meets basic competency standards. Credentialing encompasses the process of verifying qualifications, including licenses, for employment and billing purposes. Credentials are necessary to bill all insurances, including Medicare and Medicaid, even if you have your own private practice.

Credentialing is usually handled by a third party, such as HSC or FCVS, not by the state or the hospital, and verifies such information as colleges, medical schools, residency training, examinations taken and passed, medical board status, CME listings, and any legal, malpractice, or other derogatory actions that might have been taken against you. The agency provides the verifications of your DEA and PCS certification to the state medical board. You will usually also need to provide fingerprints to an outside agency. You will be responsible for the cost of these services.

I recommend that you contact your schools, training programs, and references to inform them of your applications and request that they provide the information expeditiously so that the process is not delayed. Also, if you have a medical license from other state(s), forward a copy to the new state you are applying to. This can sometimes speed up the application process.

In addition to your license, you will also need to obtain and provide your DEA certification and your state Board of Pharmacy Controlled Substance Certification. These certifications are also required before you can start practicing.

Credentials are usually re-verified every two years.

Privileging Process

The privileging process is similar to the processes for licensure and credentialing, but focuses on your experience and competency in your specialty. You must apply for privileges to provide care at an organization such as a hospital. The application must be accompanied by a range of documents that are verified by the hospital's Credentials Committee and ratified by the hospital's Medical Executive Committee. The hospital board provides final ratification of the credentialing and privileging. Information you will need to provide may include health status and vaccination records, proof of liability insurance, statement of acceptance of the bylaws and rules and regulations, and copies of your licensures, CV, and letters of recommendation. You will also need to provide case logs, especially for surgical and procedural specialists.

Applying for approval and contracts with Medicare, Medicaid, and the insurance plans in your area is usually facilitated by the organization you are joining and requires most of the information you have already supplied to get your license and facility credentials. This process can also be time-consuming, sometimes three months or more, and may contribute to a delayed start date if not completed on time.

Privileges must be renewed every two to three years as required by The Joint Commission and often the hospital's bylaws.

Types of Privileges

The hospital will provide you with a Delineation of Privileges (DOP), which lists the specific privileges you have been granted to perform. Types of privileges include:

Admitting staff privileges: Can accept patients into hospital care without needing ER approval; also called active staff privileges.

Courtesy staff privileges: Can admit a specific number of patients per year as specified in the bylaws, or visit admitted patients regarding their general medical care, but not treat them.

Consulting staff privileges: Allows specialty physicians in limited supply in the community to provide services at the request of other members of the medical staff.

Surgical staff privileges: Allow surgeons to perform operations at the hospital or an outpatient surgery facility.

Honorary staff privileges: Refers to any physician who is retired or otherwise wants to be loosely connected to a hospital without actual privileges to see or care for patients.

Refer and follow or affiliate staff privileges: Allows arranging for a patient to be admitted by a physician who has admitting privileges and allows affiliate staff to see the patient in the hospital, have access to the medical records, and directly consult with the physician in charge of the patient without being able to document in the patient's medical record.

Maintenance of Certification

Because most hospitals require board certification, if you do not maintain your certification, you may later be denied privileges until you regain your certification.

Maintenance of certification (MOC) describes programs that address continued specialty certification for physicians and provide physicians with the foundation to demonstrate lifelong learning and education. State medical boards do not require MOC.

To remain certified in their specialty, physicians must meet the continuing education requirements set by the certifying boards. Physicians can earn credit toward meeting these requirements by participating in accredited CME activities that count for MOC. Requirements vary by certifying board. In addition to the documentation of CME activities required by MOC, passing an examination/test is also required at some later time.

CHAPTER 8

Making the Move

You have chosen the practice location, have your license and credentialing/privileging, or are close to it, and have a start date. You must now find a place to live.

You likely need to make another visit to the community in which you will practice, the cost of which may or may not be covered by the organization that you are joining. Pay attention to any contract provision that stipulates how far from the hospital or healthcare organization you can live.

If you already own a home, you will need to get it on the market based on when you are moving. If you are living in an apartment, notify the apartment manager of your intended moving date.

The easiest approach is to find a rental option in the new community. Typically, you must sign a one-year lease with the provision of a financial penalty if you break the lease.

The other option is to purchase a new home or condo. With the mortgage interest rates being over 6% at the time of this writing, the monthly payments will likely be quite high, possibly making this a risky choice as you start a new practice. Some mortgage options, such as Fannie Mae, Freddie Mac, the VA, the USDA, and the FHA, allow for a lower down payment than the usual 20%.

Before your planned house or apartment hunting trip, ask someone at the organization you're joining if they can recommend a realtor in the new community whom you can contact before your visit. That way, the realtor can be prepared with several options for you to review upon arrival.

In addition, try to meet with a local banker in the new community, perhaps recommended by the organization or by the realtor you are dealing with. The banker can review your current debt structure and your starting salary to determine how much money you may be eligible to borrow toward the purchase of a new home, as well as the associated monthly payments. They can also pre-qualify you for a loan for a certain amount of money, so that you will know what price range you should be looking for in a new home.

Being pre-qualified for a loan puts you ahead of those who do not yet have a loan and are not pre-qualified, but it also puts you one step behind a cash buyer when negotiating for the new home.

If you already own a home, you don't have to sell it. Consider converting it into a rental property and using it as a long-term investment. Delay the purchase of the next home until you have saved enough money for the down payment. You will then be able to depreciate the rental property against your taxable income and pocket the rent received in excess of the loan payment. Hopefully, over time, the rental will appreciate in value if you decide to sell it, or you can keep it until it is paid off and have the full sale price as part of your retirement income.

We touched on this earlier, but it is essential to remember that you cannot begin working in your new practice until you have obtained your medical license, Board of Pharmacy license, and DEA license. If any of these requirements are not completed, you will not be able to start working, and you may not receive any compensation during this time, which can produce some serious financial distress for you and your family. So, stay very attentive to these processes during the final few months of your training.

CHAPTER 9

Transition to Attending Physician

You have received your medical license in the state that you will be practicing in, have been credentialed, and have received your privileges. You have been credited with Medicare, Medicaid, and the private insurers with whom you will be working and to whom you will be submitting bills. You are now ready to start work in your practice and at the hospital.

Before you start seeing patients, you will receive an orientation to the facility. Ideally, the orientation is in person rather than virtual, giving you an opportunity to meet the administrative staff with whom you will interact regularly. They will share details about their areas of responsibility and how what they do affects you.

You will meet people from various departments, including the medical staff office, risk management, human resources, medical records, information technology, and others. You will be trained in how to use the computer systems and programs, and will receive your login credentials for each system.

Medical Staff Bylaws

You are now an attending physician. This position brings duties, responsibilities, and potential liabilities that are considerably different from those you had as a resident or fellow. These activities are spelled out succinctly in the medical staff bylaws and rules and regulations, which you should receive as part of your orientation.

The medical staff bylaws and the rules and regulations are established by a healthcare facility or hospital to govern the behavior, responsibilities, and privileges of the medical staff, including physicians, dentists, and other healthcare professionals. These documents outline the structure and functioning of the medical staff and ensure that all members adhere to the highest standards of patient care and professional conduct.

It is essential that you read through these extensive documents early on so that you'll have a better understanding of your position as an attending physician at the hospital. The medical staff bylaws typically cover the following topics:

1. **Membership Criteria:** The qualifications and requirements for membership on the medical staff, including licensure, board certification, and professional competence.
2. **Rights and Privileges:** The rights, privileges, and responsibilities of medical staff members, such as the ability to admit and treat patients, access to hospital resources, participation in decision making, and representation on committees.
3. **Credentialing and Privileging:** The process for evaluating and approving medical staff members' qualifications, including initial credentialing, reappointment, and granting of clinical privileges based on experience, expertise, and training.
4. **Professional Conduct:** Standards of professional behavior, ethics, and code of conduct for medical staff members, including guidelines for patient interactions, confidentiality, conflict resolution, and appropriate documentation.
5. **Peer Review and Quality Improvement:** Procedures for the peer review processes, handling of complaints, and addressing disciplinary actions to ensure ongoing quality improvement and patient safety.
6. **Committee Structure:** The structure, duties, and responsibilities of various medical staff committees, such as the medical executive committee, credentials committee, pharmacy and therapeutics committee, and others.
7. **Meeting Requirements:** The frequency, format, and attendance requirements for medical staff meetings, including general meetings, department meetings, and committee meetings.

Medical staff bylaws are important for maintaining the standards of care, professionalism, and accountability within healthcare facilities. They protect patients and medical staff members and ensure a coordinated and effective healthcare delivery system.

Rules and Regulations

The medical staff rules and regulations usually cover the following topics:

1. **Admission and Discharge of Patients:** What is required of the physician in these procedures.
2. **Medical Records:** What is required for admission and discharge, as well as daily progress notes and needed procedure and surgical reports; it also specifies when notes and procedures need to be completed and on the record.
3. **General Conduct of Care:** Consent forms, administering of medications, physician availability, and response times.
4. **General Rules Regarding Surgical and Obstetrical Care:** Orders, anesthesia, care of specimens, and informed consent issues.
5. **Emergencies:** Screening, consultations, referrals, and on-call responsibilities.

For hospitals, the bylaws and rules and regulations are extensive and require substantial time to read and understand. Nevertheless, it is strongly recommended that you carefully review them prior to starting your new role as an attending physician. If you don't understand something that seems important, ask the medical staff, office personnel, or the chief of staff for clarification and explanation. Situations will likely occur that will require you to review specific passages; have them readily available in your office for review.

Hospital Quality Analysis

By this stage in your development as a physician, you have had some experience with quality metrics. You will be expected to actively participate in improving quality and safety at your hospital.

CMS has Hospital Star Ratings, which are based on a multitude of factors, many of which are physician-related, including Quality,

Safety of Care, Readmission, Patient Experience, and Timely and Effective Care.

The Leapfrog Group rates hospitals by a letter grade. Much of their scoring codes are based on physician performance, including issues of patient harm, medication safety, and healthcare-associated infections.

These systems publish their scores for public consumption and are considered important by hospital administration. Consequently, you will hear a lot about these quality rating programs at department meetings, quality meetings, and meetings of the Medical Executive Committee (MEC).

As you start practicing at the hospital, your patient care will be closely evaluated by the quality department under Focused Professional Practice Evaluation (FPPE). The specific areas of your practice that are followed are determined by the MEC per specialty and usually extend for the first few cases or procedures. Later, FPPE may be triggered by unanticipated outcomes or poor peer review.

Assuming you have passed the FPPE process, the Ongoing Professional Practice Evaluation (OPPE) process is activated after about six months. Often, an outside company follows metrics such as the hospital-reported complication rate, mortality rate, readmission rate, and other parameters. Those physicians not meeting the required parameters may be placed on FPPE for the delinquent areas. The MEC then decides the next steps, and a performance improvement plan (PIP) is developed for the physician.

CHAPTER 10

Coding, Billing, and Driving Revenue

Most organizations that you join have their own professional coding and billing specialists or contract with an outside agency. Still, it is important that you understand the basics of this process because you play a critical role in ensuring that you are paid for the services that you render. The organization may arrange for you to receive basic education in the coding process as you start working.

Basics of Coding and Billing

To bill Medicare, Medicaid, or a health insurance entity, you must have an NPI (National Provider Identifier) number. The NPI is a unique 10-digit numerical identifier assigned to individual providers or healthcare entities. Providers, employers, health plans, and payers use these numbers for billing purposes. Covered healthcare providers and all health plans and healthcare clearinghouses must use the NPI in the administrative and financial transactions adopted under HIPAA (Health Insurance Portability and Accountability Act). You can apply for an NPI number at the NPI registry: npps.cms.hhs.gov.

The billing process begins with the appointment. The patient is asked to provide information about themselves and their insurance. If necessary, the front office personnel will ensure that they have received the appropriate referrals for the patient.

The next step, your examination of the patient and subsequent report, is the most critical aspect of the coding and billing process. You must document in considerable detail the reason the patient came to visit you, the elements of the physical examination, and the medical decision-making that went into your treatment plan.

The current requirement is that each service include "a medically appropriate history and or examination." The more information you include in your report, the easier it is for coders and billers to be accurate and to ensure payment for your services.

You will provide the codes for each procedure, or somebody in the organization will do it for you. The code for the procedure will then be referred to a biller who will ensure that all the necessary information for the code is included. The coding and billing information will then be sent to the payer. If the biller or payer determines that information is missing, they will contact you and request that you provide the needed information.

You must address any payer questions or concerns promptly in order to ensure timely payment. This part of the process sometimes takes three or more months to complete.

Types of Codes

The main types of medical codes used in coding and billing are ICD codes, CPT codes, and HCPCS codes.

- **ICD (International Classification of Diseases)** codes are used to document diagnoses and are the global standard for diagnostic codes. ICD-10 stands for the International Classification of Diseases, 10th edition. These codes have been developed by the World Health Organization and adopted by governments around the world. In the United States, there are two types of ICD-10 systems: ICD-10-CM (clinical modification) is used for diagnosis, and ICD-10-PCS (procedure coding system) is used for inpatient hospital procedures.
- **CPT (Current Procedural Terminology)** codes are used to document medical procedures and are primarily used for billing purposes. These codes capture the physician's and other clinical services delivered and connect the services with the code for billing.
- **HCPCS (Healthcare Common Procedure Coding System)** codes are used for services, procedures, and supplies not covered by CPT codes, such as ambulance services, drugs, and durable medical equipment.

The codes that you will deal with most often are the CPT codes for evaluation and management (EM). These codes, which vary for new patients and established patients, address such medically appropriate history and/or examination, along with medical decision-making. The codes vary with the level of medical decision-making and the time allotted.

For physicians who perform procedures and/or operations, there are CPT codes specific to a particular procedure or operation. They are very detailed as to exactly what was done during the procedure and are selected based on what is written in your procedure or operative report.

Billing for Services

Based on the information that you submit in your report, including the appropriate history, physical examination, and time involved, a billing specialist or an outside agency will generate a bill to send to the appropriate payer. In some cases, the bill will be broken down into the amount the insurance company is responsible for covering and the amount the patient is responsible for paying.

This process may change as artificial intelligence is incorporated into the computerized medical record. AI may eventually be used to develop a record of the patient-physician conversation and discussion, and may be able to generate a visit code and bill based on the information included in the medical record.

When the payer receives the medical record, codes, and bill, they decide whether to pay the bill or to dispute it. If they dispute it, they will send your organization the specific reason for the dispute, at which point you may be contacted to explain in more detail why the code and bill are as they are. A key takeaway is that if something is not written in the record, it is difficult to dispute a denial of charge. In rare circumstances, there may be an allegation of fraud, which then raises the dispute to a much higher level.

As you can see, coding and billing are complicated and sometimes confusing. Almost all organizations have trained professionals who implement and oversee this process. You, the physician, do not need to know all the intricacies of the process, just the basics.

For more detailed information, the books and references listed in Appendix G are excellent resources.

CHAPTER 11

Financial Considerations as You Start Your Practice

As you start your new practice, your pay will increase substantially; it may be three to five times more than what you were making during your training. This salary increase often triggers a desire to purchase things for the house, for your family, and for yourself that you may have been putting off for the past several years. However, there are other significant financial considerations that you must be aware of and address during this transition period. (These topics are well covered in the May 2024 and May 2025 issues of Kiplinger Personal Finance magazine.)

As you start your practice, consider these guidelines:

Set up and Stick to a Budget: A solid budget provides a clear picture of where your money is going, allowing you to identify areas where you can decrease spending and dedicate more funds to wealth-creation goals. You can do this by reviewing your spending over the past year or more. You typically can access your spending history for free through your credit card company or bank. This may not provide a comprehensive view; however, you may want to consider using an app such as Monarch Money or Copilot Money to get a more detailed picture of your spending habits.

A couple of rules of thumb for spending, according to Investopedia, include limiting your housing costs to no more than 32% of your net income and your car-related expenses to around 10%. It is also recommended that you keep your split between groceries and restaurants at about 50-50. You also need to consider "extras" you value, such as vacations or hobbies, and determine what percentage of your income to spend on those categories.

Finally, evaluate where you can trim spending if necessary. You should also review your budget expenses regularly, ideally on a monthly basis.

Pay off Student Loans and Other Debts: Many physicians finish their training with debts of more than $200,000 from student loans and living expenses over the past 11 years or more. Many probably have federal education loans with fixed interest rates, so changes in short-term interest rates nationally won't affect current payments.

Of greater significance is credit card debt because of the high interest rates on outstanding balances — now in the vicinity of 25%. You can reduce these interest rates by transferring your outstanding balance to a less costly credit card account. Several card issuers are offering 0% interest rates on balance transfers for anywhere from 12 to 21 months, so that while you are paying off your debt, the interest is not increasing the amount that you owe. Pay off the balance during the 0% interest period.

If you are unable to meet the requirements for these transfers, ask your credit card company for a better deal where the average reduction is in the vicinity of 6%. Also, it is worth considering an automatic payment from your bank account to the loan servicer. This ensures that your payments arrive on time, which avoids late fees and contributes to a positive credit history.

Set Up and Fund an Emergency Account: Your life can be derailed by a sudden or unexpected unemployment, a serious health condition, or a natural disaster. Set up an emergency savings account that covers three to six months' worth of regular expenses. This is money you can't afford to lose and should be invested in an easily accessible savings account or money market deposit account.

Open a 401(k) Account and Invest Fully Each Year: Most large healthcare organizations automatically enroll workers in their 401(k) plans. Currently, you can contribute up to $23,000 in a 401(k) and other employer-sponsored plans on an annual basis. Contributions are tax-deferred if you invest in a traditional 401(k), but withdrawals are taxed when taken. With a Roth 401(k), if available, contributions are made with after-tax dollars, but withdrawals are tax-free in retirement. In many cases, employers offer matching contributions up to a certain percentage of what you invest.

Consider Insurance Options: Most healthcare organizations provide health insurance options and disability insurance. Although disability insurance may be offered as part of your employment package, it is worth considering obtaining your own policy outside of the organization. For a young physician, the rates are generally quite low and do not increase as you age. The disability payments from the employer-sponsored plan may not be enough to cover your family expenses if you become disabled. A private plan will help cover these costs should they become necessary.

Life insurance may or may not be part of the package you're offered. Consider buying a term policy, not a whole life policy, large enough to pay off all the debts as well as provide funds for a spouse to invest, to maintain a good lifestyle, educate the kids, etc. The younger the age at which the policy is purchased, the cheaper the premiums and the lower the likelihood of a health condition that would make the insurance difficult to obtain.

Other insurance options, such as auto insurance, homeowners insurance, and umbrella insurance, are not typically offered but are important for you to consider. Auto insurance is usually required by the state. Obtaining a homeowners' insurance policy is generally recommended to cover your home and its contents should a disaster occur. Note that flood insurance is not covered by a standard homeowners' insurance policy.

Umbrella insurance provides coverage if your homeowners or auto insurance claims exceed the liability limits of your existing policies. Such coverage is beneficial if you have significant assets or are vulnerable to exhausting your standard policies.

Get Help from a Professional Financial Adviser: A certified financial planner (CFP) can provide guidance as you move forward in your practice. Look for an adviser who is a fiduciary, which means the individual must look out for your best interest above his or her own. All certified financial planners are required to adhere to fiduciary standards, so limiting your search to CFPs is a good place to start.

Costs for these services vary and can be quite high. A fee-only planner charges only for the advice given. Some financial advisers charge by a method known as assets under management (AUM), which bases fees on a percentage of the value of your portfolio. In other cases, you may be charged on an hourly basis for the services provided and have no additional expenses above this.

Sometimes, if you have investments with an organization, financial planners are available to you at little or no cost. I encourage you to investigate these services early on with the expectation that they can help you considerably with investments into the future.

Recognized financial adviser Suze Orman has some sound financial advice for younger people in the early stages of their work careers: ***Live below your means, but within your needs.***

Living below your means is choosing not to spend every penny you make but to spend only what is necessary to meet your needs. This could mean living with a roommate or living in a less expensive part of town. It can also mean buying a less expensive used car with a low down payment and low monthly payments.

Spending above your means can lead to excessive debt and leave you unprepared for an emergency. Even as your income increases, you should continue to live below your means. It sets you up for financial success for the rest of your life.

CHAPTER 12

Work-Life Balance vs. Burnout

By now, you have mastered much of the maze of becoming a practicing physician and have started your practice. Your office location, exam rooms, and staff have been determined, and your office is outfitted. You have agreed on the office hours, number of patients to be seen daily, and/or your overall productivity. You have a place to live, and your income is assured.

You have been working hard up to this point, but always under the supervision and direction of people above you. Now you have more control, but not total control. You will be seeing patients, but you will also need to update the electronic medical record daily and respond to phone calls, text messages, and emails from patients. If you have hospital privileges, you will need to set aside time for routine hospital-related activities as well as urgent situations that may arise with your hospitalized patients. Also, you will need to spend time on prior authorizations and insurance company requests for additional information about a particular patient.

It is likely that there will be many interruptions during the day: committee assignments, office meetings, and hospital meetings. You must still answer to the organization's administrators, who will closely monitor your performance in terms of quality of care and financial aspects.

That's just your professional life. In addition, you may be married and have or plan to start a family. Your life outside the practice includes shopping, cleaning and laundry, and childcare. You also cannot neglect the fact that you need appropriate sleep and exercise, as well as healthcare for yourself and your family. You must be prepared for the unexpected, such as health concerns, injuries, transportation issues, and other situations that will require your time away from work.

Your Work-Life Balance

Now is the time to consider your work-life balance. It is essential to recognize that these two domains are not distinct but are likely to be interwoven, and their boundaries are often blurred. Especially today, with the presence of cell phones, beepers, and computers, it is common for work activities to spill over into leisure time.

Don't assume that a balance will develop between work and life; this is not usually the case. Instead, creating a balance takes thought and some effort. Consider developing a work-life budget. Identify how you are currently spending your time. Set goals to identify long-term objectives. Then track your results to see how you are doing.

1. **Keep a log of your activities and the time spent on each for a week or more.** Separate out the time you spend into categories, such as direct patient care, clerical tasks, administrative tasks, academic work, education time, social activities, family, friends, exercise, sleeping, and errands. Also look at how much time you spend doing work tasks away from work, such as checking on patients by phone, monitoring email, and doing academic administrative work at home. Then, map out your annual time spent in each category, including vacation days.
2. **Set career goals.** These goals could be short-term, mid-range, and long-term. Take into account the expectations of administrators, partners, patients, family, and self. Focus on what you would like to achieve in each area, such as the number of work relative value units for the upcoming year.

   Designate a time allocation for each activity, such as time for clinic, returning patient phone calls, reviewing data, preparing for surgery, etc. Also consider other activities that you might want to be involved in, such as hospital administration, societal activities, and committees.
3. **Set personal goals.** Include the time you commit to family, personal health, exercise, spiritual health, and seeing your doctor or dentist. Also, budget for the unexpected, including illnesses and other life obstacles.

4. **Stick to your budget as much as possible.** If you have allocated time for non-work activities, let your partners, office, and staff know, and then try to get away. Sometimes it is necessary to carefully allocate your time, and at other times it is necessary to just say no.

Studies show that when physicians identify the aspect of their work that they find meaningful and perform that part at least 20% of the time, they are far less likely to burn out than those who do not do so. Being aware of work-life balance can improve career satisfaction.

Work-life balance is not static. Determining the right course for you and assessing your goals is an ongoing process, constantly changing to accommodate new needs, goals, and situations. Maintaining your work-life balance demands your constant attention and should remain on your "to-do" list at all times.

Avoiding Burnout

Because physicians feel the need to be available to their patients at all times, it is not unusual to become overwhelmed by phone calls, texts, and emails, as well as insurance company, hospital, and office demands. Other factors that can lead to stress and depression, precursors to burnout, include:

- Number of nights on call per week.
- Number of hours worked per week.
- Compensation determined entirely based on billings or other metrics.
- Loss of autonomy in how to spend time.
- Time spent on computer documentation.
- Lack of adequate staffing help.
- Pressure and lack of support from administrative staff.
- Fear of malpractice claims.

Physician burnout is a state of emotional, physical, and mental exhaustion that results from prolonged and excessive stress in the medical profession. It can lead to feelings of detachment, decreased empathy for patients, reduced job performance, and overall dissatisfaction with work and life. Burnout can negatively impact patient care, leading to medical errors and poor patient outcomes. It can also result in higher rates of attrition in the healthcare workforce. According to reported studies, more than half of the nation's physicians are experiencing burnout, and this number appears to be increasing.

Addressing these issues on a personal level as well as on the healthcare system level requires several strategies.

From a personal perspective, strategies include:

1. **Mindfulness and Stress Management.** Practicing mindfulness techniques such as meditation, yoga, or deep breathing exercises can reduce stress and improve emotional well-being.
2. **Cognitive Behavioral Therapy (CBT).** Engaging with a mental health professional to explore thoughts and feelings can address negative thought patterns and develop coping strategies.
3. **Physical Activity.** Make time for regular exercise that includes aerobic activity and weight training. This has been shown to improve energy levels, clear the mind, and provide health benefits when continued over time.
4. **Nutrition and Sleep.** Maintaining a healthy diet and ensuring adequate sleep can improve physical and mental health, helping combat burnout.
5. **A Work-Life Budget.** As described above, trying to create a work-life balance can stave off burnout.

See Appendix H for burnout causes according to Medscape.

While practicing medicine will occupy most of your days and many of your nights, you should take into consideration other important aspects of life that need to be addressed. If you have children, it is important that you spend time with them doing the things that they like to do and supporting them in their activities, such as sporting events. Many times, they will need your attention with their schoolwork, especially at home in the evenings. It may be difficult to accomplish this after a long day of work, but it is essential that you make time for them. The same applies to your spouse or partner.

Make time for yourself. Take up a hobby. Learn to play a musical instrument, paint, or speak a new language. Learn ballroom dancing or join a hiking club. These activities will give you personal pleasure and take your mind off the medical duties of the day.

Seeking Help

Some issues associated with depression and burnout cannot be handled by you alone; you need involvement from the organization's administrative staff.

To help decrease burnout among staff, organizations can:

1. Give more autonomy to the clinicians in the control of their work hours and productivity requirements.
2. Develop a community support network of psychology practitioners and establish a physician well-being committee to address the physicians and their issues, and try to resolve them wherever possible.
3. Include physicians on the Information Technology Committee to help streamline the EMR with such things as ambient listening and AI responses to texts, calls, and emails.
4. Increase staffing and support in the office environment to make the office activities smoother, faster, and more efficient.
5. Allow and encourage physicians to use all their vacation (PTO) time without financial penalties when they return.

If you have made the recommended changes to your work-life balance, and if the organization has not been forthcoming in making changes to your work requirements, it may be necessary to take drastic steps to address your burnout. I encourage you to consider other paths as discussed earlier in the book.

If you are in a primary care situation, consider going out on your own as a concierge physician and report to nobody but yourself. Consider retraining in another specialty that does not entail emergencies and night calls. Also consider physician-related side gigs, such as insurance company chart review, working with attorneys in malpractice cases, telehealth, teaching or research, and a physician ombudsman, helping patients navigate the healthcare system for a fee.

If none of these activities appeals to you, it may be time to pursue a completely different line of work outside of medicine. There is no simple answer or easy treatment to resolve issues of work-life balance and burnout. It takes a concerted effort to make the changes necessary to decrease work-life imbalance and burnout.

Reclaiming the Joy of Medicine: Finding Purpose, Fulfillment, and Happiness in Today's Medical Industry by Alen Voskanian raises several points for you to consider as you work through feelings of burnout:

- "Always do the right thing for your patients, no matter what. If you work at a place that doesn't allow you to do the right thing, it's time to find another place."
- "Comparison and competition might have helped you get into a good school or land a good job, but now you must let it go. Like a double-edged sword, it will always make you feel less than others and exhaust you emotionally."
- "Seek care when sick, and don't be afraid to call in sick. Ask for help when you need it. Others want to be helpful. Don't allow shame or stigma prevent you from seeking help when you need it."
- "Make time for your loved ones. If or when you have children, never miss their graduations, recitals, and birthday parties. These are not little things. These are the big things that matter."
- "Prioritize your health and well-being. Pay attention to your nutrition, sleep, exercise, and mind."
- "Practice gratitude."
- "Curb your enthusiasm for perfection. Sometimes good enough is the right choice."
- "When you lose your way and can't remember why you do what you do, remind yourself of your purpose for going into healthcare. If you feel separated from your purpose, find your way back."

- "Read and reread this list periodically to remind yourself that your joy is yours."
- "Having joy is your right. You deserve it, your family deserves it, and your patients deserve it. If you have lost your joy in medicine, reclaim it!"

CHAPTER 13

Social Media Pros and Cons

Thousands of current and potential patients use internet websites and social media to gather medical information, check symptoms and treatment, and research potential physicians. The medical information they obtain may be inaccurate or even completely false. Realize that potential and current patients may also be researching you! Your organization will typically add a picture of you on its official website, as well as information about your training, subspecialty interest, and skills, and possibly even your awards and accomplishments. Check this site periodically to ensure accuracy. Also, as you begin your practice, put your name in the search bar of your internet browser and see what information comes up.

After you have begun seeing patients, they may provide reviews of you and your organization on such sites as HealthGrades, ZocDoc, and RateMDs. Check these sites periodically to see what patients are saying about you and use their comments to help you improve your practice style and methods.

Social media websites such as Facebook, X, LinkedIn, YouTube, TikTok, and Instagram often include discussions and videos about medical information. As noted previously, much of this medical information is inaccurate and can sometimes lead patients to make incorrect decisions about their health.

Some organizations have policies about physicians using social media to discuss medical issues, and you need to be aware of these policies before you post any medical information on these sites. It is also important that you not post any information about a patient or information that can be easily traced back to a specific patient. Failure to maintain confidentiality could land you in considerable legal trouble.

CHAPTER 14

Keeping Abreast of Challenges and Changes

Healthcare is changing rapidly. Many hospitals are closing or limiting their service lines due to financial constraints. This is especially problematic in rural areas where many hospitals are forced to close. If you are employed by a hospital in danger of closing, you will be expected to increase productivity. And certainly, if the hospital closes your line of practice or closes completely, this will have a significant impact on you and your practice.

Private Equity in Healthcare

Many medical practices and hospitals are being acquired by private equity organizations that then assume ownership. These organizations are primarily motivated by profit; quality is not a significant consideration, although they may proclaim that it is. A fairly standard model of private equity is to buy an organization, focus on maximizing profits for a period of time, and then, after five or six years, sell the organization to another private equity firm for a profit. Consequently, there's considerable pressure on physicians and their practices to increase their productivity by seeing more patients and performing more procedures.

The productivity requirements that negatively affect the doctor-patient relationship are driving some doctors into private practice.

Telehealth

Telehealth gained in popularity during the pandemic. CMS and many insurance carriers agreed to pay for this service at about the same rates as a face-to-face encounter. Many patients have found this to be beneficial, as it saves them considerable time and effort, especially for routine visits.

Recognizing that telehealth companies can take patients away from their practices, many physicians are incorporating telehealth into their daily practice. If you have not already done so, you might want to consider incorporating some aspect of telehealth into your new practice.

Unionization

In some parts of the country, particularly in larger cities with more extensive physician groups, unionization is becoming a topic of discussion because physicians feel as though they have lost control of the practice of medicine to the administrators who are making all the decisions and requiring more productivity from their physicians. Some organizations have physician advisory groups, but they usually have little or no voice in or control over what the upper-level administrators determine is necessary to produce the required profit.

The best way for physicians to advocate for themselves is to join forces with other physicians nationwide. The American Medical Association (AMA) represents all physicians and is active in advocating for its members. In addition, most medical specialties have their own societies that support their members in dealing with insurers and government agencies about issues such as increasing pay for services, fixing prior authorizations, and reducing physician burnout.

There is a cost associated with joining these organizations, but your membership can prove valuable personally and professionally.

CHAPTER 15

The New Frontier of AI

One of the more significant changes in the practice of medicine is the use of artificial intelligence. The American Medical Association (AMA) typically uses the term "augmented intelligence" when referring to artificial intelligence in the context of medicine, highlighting AI's role as an assistive technology that enhances human intelligence rather than replaces it. The term underscores the importance of physicians and other healthcare professionals remaining at the center of patient care, with AI tools serving to support their decision-making and improve efficiency.

In healthcare, AI can:

1. Highlight the most important and relevant aspects of a patient–physician conversation.
2. Extract data from the patient's medical records that can be valuable to guide treatment.
3. Decrease administrative paperwork burdens, allowing physicians to see more patients.
4. Facilitate insurance approvals.
5. Summarize large amounts of information about patients that come from referrals.
6. Leverage available registry data for research in a much more effective and efficient way.
7. Gather information about symptoms, diagnoses, and treatments. A shortcoming of this type of AI is that it is general rather than patient-specific.

Enhanced AI in Healthcare

An emerging and potentially more useful type of AI is CAI, or clinical augmented intelligence. CAI enhances the benefits of AI by adding patient-specific information to provide individualized recommendations for the patient. This minimizes the physician's time in reviewing prior reports and patient information and allows time for more personal contact with the patient.

While CAI is still an emerging technology, several AI programs are currently available to assist physicians and patients alike.

Ambient Listening. Ambient listening programs such as NextGen Ambient Assist convert patient-provider conversations into a structured note that can quickly be reviewed and sent into the patient's chart. These notes can then be converted into actual billing codes, saving the office staff considerable time. Practices that use this tool have found it to be a major time saver.

AI Agents. Agentforce, from Salesforce, incorporates AI "agents" that can alleviate administrative burdens and improve patient communications while giving providers the space to focus on complex cases that demand their expertise.

A patient has access to an AI agent that reaches out to check on them after a procedure, reminding them to follow up on test results, and asking them if they have any unexpected reactions that need to be addressed. The agent monitors patient progress and even reschedules labs or appointments as needed, all while maintaining a detailed understanding of the patient's medical history and ongoing treatment.

Enhanced Communication. In some locations, AI is being used to respond to patient texts and emails requesting answers to their questions or concerns. These answers are based on information in the patients' medical charts. The physician must review the response for accuracy before it is sent; however, the preliminary work done by the AI program saves the physician much time and facilitates a timely response.

An April 2023 *JAMA Internal Medicine* article reports that patients are more positive about the AI chatbot responses than those from the physician because the responses appear to me more empathetic and complete.

Imaging Review. AI is also used in several specialties, including radiology, pathology, dermatology, and ophthalmology, to view images and provide a review of the study, including the positive and negative findings. It is also being used in telehealth to evaluate data from patient monitors, which can be extensive and require a significant amount of time for review by the physician.

General Information. Increasingly, patients turn to AI tools online like ChatGPT and Gemini to evaluate their symptoms, read about their diagnoses, and learn about types of treatment for their conditions. AI is not perfect, however, and the information provided can be incomplete, inaccurate, or out of date. There is also the danger of hallucinations and confabulations, meaning the AI tool makes up information without any basis in research or fact.

If the patient comes in with misinformation gleaned from the internet, it is important that you, as the medical expert, correct them and give them appropriate information and guidance.

Looking to the Future

As AI advances, there must be collaboration among clinicians, technology developers, and regulatory bodies to ensure secure, reliable, and fully integrated processes for clinical workflows.

We must ensure AI safety, including appropriate clinical, technical, and administrative governance policies, risk management procedures, people, and technologies to ensure that AI is monitored and its use is safe, secure, effective, private, ethical, and equitable. Healthcare organizations must create policies and procedures to ensure that patients and clinicians are aware, when possible, that AI-enabled systems are being used for clinical and administrative decision-making and communication. We can position AI as an enhancement to care, not a replacement for it, effectively balancing innovation with the human connection at the heart of healthcare.

The shared goal must be to harness AI in a way that truly enhances the quality of care, supports our clinicians, and fosters lasting trust with the patients we treat. The Trustworthy and Responsible AI Network (TRAIN) is a consortium to facilitate safe and effective AI adoption in the United States and in Europe. The purpose is to serve as a practical network of health system stakeholders focused on advancing responsible health AI. It supports healthcare organizations in implementing health AI in a trustworthy and responsible manner to improve healthcare across diverse settings and populations.

CHAPTER 16

Physician Side Gigs: Opportunities for Additional Income

Under the weight of medical school debt and the high cost of living, some physicians look for ways to supplement their income outside of their regular medical practice. Some of these activities relate to medicine, such as disability and file review, independent medical examination, expert witness practice, and utilization review. Other "side gigs" include product development, medical communications, research, teaching, and writing. (See Appendix I for information on physician side gigs.)

One area outside of medicine that attracts physicians is real estate investing. In a recent poll of 3,500 physicians, 37% said real estate investing is their preferred side gig, according to Op-Med. It is attractive because it provides real property, tax benefits, and consistent cash flow without a full-time commitment. Another side gig outside of medicine is day trading on the stock market. This requires close attention to be successful and may intrude on daily medical practice.

Some other side gigs that involve medicine are *locum tenens* and moonlighting. *Locum tenens* can be lucrative, but it may be difficult to fit into your current job, and it takes you away from home and family for extended periods. Moonlighting time is usually added to your already busy schedule and takes you away from family and leisure activities, although it may pay well. The extra work and time away from family may lead to burnout, so it should be carefully thought out. Note that some contracts for your primary employment may preclude your opportunity to moonlight.

The American Association for Physician Leadership (physicianleaders.org) published two books by Sylvie Stacy, MD, MPH, on the topic of alternative careers for physicians: *50 Nonclinical Careers for Physicians* and *50 Unconventional Clinical Careers for Physicians*. They are available on the AAPL website (https://www.physicianleaders.org/publications/books).

SEAK (www.seak.com) is an organization that provides skills, education, abilities, and knowledge (SEAK) to help physicians find supplemental work. They provide seminars on topics such as expert witness training and practice, disability and file review, and independent medical examination practice.

EPILOGUE

I hope that you have found this handbook to be useful as you complete your residency or fellowship and begin your practice of medicine. As you can see, there are many crucial steps that you must take in what can be a long and arduous process. Take each step carefully and with deep consideration, as it will significantly facilitate your process.

Although the process is difficult, it is worth the time and effort. And, if done carefully and with due consideration, it will make your life as a physician much easier and more enjoyable for you and your family.

I hope you never lose sight of the goodness you are fostering in the care of your patients. Never forget the benefits you are bestowing on your patients by giving them your best advice and care.

EPILOGUE

APPENDICES

Appendix A
Physician Recruiting Firms

- Alpha Apex Group
  https://www.alphaapexgroup.com
- AMN Healthcare
  https://www.amnhealthcare.com
- Arthur Marshall
  https://www.arthurmarshall.com
- Careers by KevinMD
  https://www.healthecareers.com/kevinmd/search-jobs
- CompHealth
  https://comphealth.com
- Indeed
  www.indeed.com
- JAMA Career Center
  https://careers.jamanetwork.com
- Physicians Thrive
  https://physiciansthrive.com
- Practice Link
  https://www.practicelink.com
- US Acute Care Solutions
  https://www.usacs.com
- Weatherby Healthcare
  https://weatherbyhealthcare.com

Appendix B

Physician Locums Firms

- AMN Healthcare
  https://www.amnhealthcare.com/staffing/physician/locums/
- Barton Associates
  https://www.bartonassociates.com
- Caliber Healthcare Solutions
  https://www.caliberhealth.com/
- CompHealth
  https://comphealth.com
- Crawford Thomas
  https://www.crawfordthomas.com
- Elite365
  https://elite365.com/locum-tenens-staffing/
- Global Medical Staffing
  https://gmedical.com/
- Hayes Locums
  https://www.hayeslocums.com/
- Interim Physicians
  https://www.interimphysicians.com/
- Jackson + Coker Locum Tenens
  https://jacksoncoker.com/healthcare-staffing-solutions/locum-tenens-staffing/
- LocumJobsOnline
  https://www.locumjobsonline.com/jobs
- Locum Tenens USA
  https://locumtenensusa.com/
- LocumTenens.com
  https://www.locumtenens.com/
- Locumpedia
  https://www.locumpedia.com

- MASC Medical Recruitment Firm
  https://mascmedical.com/
- Physician Resources, Inc. (PRI)
  https://physicianresources.com/
- Vista Staffing
  https://www.vistastaff.com/
- Weatherby Healthcare
  https://weatherbyhealthcare.com

Appendix C

Best and Worst States for Physician Practice

Montana, South Dakota, and Nebraska are the top three states for physicians to practice in the U.S., according to WalletHub's 2024 ranking published in March. Hawaii, Rhode Island and New Jersey were deemed the worst.

The annual ranking is based on two key dimensions: opportunity-competition and medical environment. Within those dimensions, WalletHub evaluated 19 metrics, including average annual wage, number of hospitals per capita, quality of the public health system, and hospital safety grades. Each of the 19 metrics was graded on a 100-point scale, with 100 representing the most favorable conditions for physicians. WalletHub used the average across all 19 metrics to calculate an overall score.

The Nine Best States for Physicians:

1. Montana
2. South Dakota
3. Nebraska
4. Utah
5. Indiana
6. Minnesota
7. Wisconsin
8. Idaho
9. Iowa

The 16 Worst States for Physicians

1. Hawaii
2. Rhode Island
3. New Jersey
4. Massachusetts
5. New York
6. New Mexico
7. District of Columbia
8. Oregon

9. Illinois
10. Alaska
11. Delaware
12. Arkansas
13. Pennsylvania
14. Maryland
15. Florida
16. West Virginia

Three more notes from the ranking:

- Montana, which ranked No. 1 overall, placed first for opportunity and competition and third for medical environment.
- Nebraska (No. 3 overall) ranked first for medical environment and 22nd for opportunity and rank.
- Hawaii placed 49th for opportunity and rank and 47th for medical environment.

Appendix D
Major Physician Employers

- Permanente Medical Group
- Optum Inc
- Piedmont Healthcare
- HCA Healthcare
- Vanderbilt Health
- Ascension
- Brigham and Women's Hospital
- Cleveland Clinic-HealthCare Partners IPA
- Northwell Health
- Mayo Foundation for Medical Education and Research
- Beaumont Health
- Advocate Aurora Health
- NYU Langone Hospitals

Appendix E

Law Firms and Other Organizations that Specialize in Physician Contracting

National Law Firms Specializing in Physician Contracting

These firms have a nationwide presence and are recognized for expertise in physician employment agreements, including negotiation, review, compliance with Stark Law and Anti-Kickback Statute, and related healthcare transactions.

- **Bass, Berry & Sims, PLC**
  bassberry.com
- **Buchanan Ingersoll & Rooney, PC**
  bipc.com
- **Crowell & Moring, LLP**
  crowell.com
- **Duane Morris, LLP**
  duanemorris.com
- **Epstein Becker Green, PC**
  ebglaw.com
- **Hall Render Killian Heath & Lyman, PC**
  hallrender.com
- **King & Spalding, LLP**
  kslaw.com
- **McDermott Will & Emery, LLP**
  mwe.com
- **Nixon Peabody, LLP**
  nixonpeabody.com
- **Sheppard Mullin Richter & Hampton, LLP**
  sheppardmullin.com

Specialized Firms and Boutiques Focused on Physician Contracts

These are smaller or niche firms/boutiques with a strong emphasis on physician employment reviews, often at fixed fees, and tailored to individual doctors or groups.

- **Concierge Healthcare Attorneys, LLC**
  conciergehealthcareattorneysllc.com
- **Contract Rx®**
  mycontractrx.com
- Hendershot Cowart, PC
  https://www.hchlawyers.com/
- **Physician Agreements Health Law**
  pahealthlaw.com
- **Physicians' Advocates℠**
  physiciansadvocates.com
- **Resolve**
  www.resolve.com/attorneys
- **The Holloman Law Group (HLG)**
  hollomanlawgroup.com

Contact state medical associations for additional local referrals.

Other resources:

- Contract Diagnostics: contractdiagnostics.com
- Physicians Thrive: physiciansthrive.com
- AMA Physicians Guide to Hospital Employment Contracts: ama-assn.org

Appendix F
Physician Salary Ranges by Specialty

The 20 Specialties with the Highest Average Compensation

Neurosurgery	$749,140
Thoracic Surgery	$689,969
Orthopaedic Surgery	$679,517
Pediatric (Gen) Surgery	$647,721
Plastic Surgery	$621,445
Oral & Maxillofacial Surgery	$616,748
Radiation Oncology	$588,678
Cardiology	$587,360
Vascular Surgery	$576,452
Interventional Radiology	$572,617
Radiology	$571,749
Urology	$559,474
Gastroenterology	$537,870
Otolaryngology ENT	$523,369
Anesthesiology	$523,277
Dermatology	$508,401
Oncology	$502,465
Colon & Rectal Surgery	$487,085
General Surgery	$482,574
Ophthalmology	$477,232

The 20 Specialties with the Lowest Average Annual Compensation

Pediatric Endocrinology	$230,426
Pediatric Rheumatology	$231,574
Pediatric Infectious Disease	$248,322
Pediatric Hematology & Oncology	$255,733
Medical Genetics	$259,564

- Pediatric Nephrology $263,013
- Pediatrics $265,230
- Pediatric Pulmonology $282,000
- Child Neurology $289,738
- Endocrinology $290,606
- Geriatrics $291,968
- Medicine/Pediatrics $296, 665
- Pediatric Gastroenterology $298,457
- Allergy & Immunology $308,846
- Preventive Medicine $310,177
- Pediatric Emergency Medicine $312,271
- Family Medicine $318,959
- Infectious Disease $320,730
- Rheumatology $324,954
- Internal Medicine $326,116

Source: Doximity. Physician Compensation Report 2025. https://www.doximity.com/reports/physician-compensation-report/2025

Appendix G
Coding Books and References

Core Medical Coding Reference Books

These are the primary official codebooks used by physicians for billing and documentation, and by AAPC-certified coders (e.g., CPC for physician office coding) for accurate claim submission. These codebooks are published annually by the American Medical Association (AMA) or the Centers for Medicare & Medicaid Services (CMS), with 2024 editions currently on sale as of October 2025.

- **ICD-10-CM 2024: The Complete Official Codebook**
  Official diagnosis coding guidelines from the CDC/CMS, essential for all coders and physicians to classify patient conditions and symptoms.
- **CPT 2024 Professional Edition**
  AMA's official procedural coding book with guidelines and rules, the gold standard for outpatient physician services; includes E/M documentation rules critical for AAPC CPC certification.
- **HCPCS Level II Professional 2024**
  Complete official codebook for non-physician services, supplies, and drugs (e.g., Medicare billing); required for comprehensive coding in physician practices.
- **ICD-10-PCS 2024: The Complete Official Codebook**
  Official procedural coding for inpatient hospital settings (CMS); used by coders for facility-based procedures, though less common in pure physician office workflows.

Additional Coding Tools

- Codingintel.com
- Codify by AAPC
- Procedure Desk Reference (2025 eBook): AAPC's procedural coding companion with quick-reference tools for CPT application in physician services.

Appendix H

Burnout Causes and Percentages (Medscape 2024)

- Too many bureaucratic tasks — charting, paperwork: 60%
- Too many hours at work: 40%
- Lack of respect from administrators/employers: 40%
- Insufficient compensation: 38%
- Lack of control/autonomy: 32%
- Computerization of practice (EHRs): 23%
- Lack of respect from patients: 22%
- Government regulations: 13%
- Other: 9%

Appendix I
Resources for Physician Side Gigs

- *50 Nonclinical Careers for Physicians: Fulfilling, Meaningful, and Lucrative Alternatives to Direct Patient Care*, by Sylvie Stacy, MD, MPH. AAPL. https://www.physicianleaders.org/publications/books/50-nonclinical-careers-for-physicians-fulfilling-meaningful-and-lucrative-alternatives-to-direct-patient-care.
- *50 Unconventional Clinical Careers for Physicians: Unique Ways to Use Your Medical Degree Without Leaving Patient Care*, by Sylvie Stacy, MD, MPH. AAPL. https://www.physicianleaders.org/publications/books/50-unconventional-clinical-careers-for-physicians-unique-ways-to-use-your-medical-degree-without-leaving-patient-care-stacy?v=42790329024692
- Nonclinical Careers for Physicians Self-Study. AAPL. https://www.physicianleaders.org/education/course/non-clinical-careers-for-physicians.
- Physician Side Gigs Newsletter. https://www.physiciansidegigs.com.
- Top Side Gigs for Physicians. Sermo. https://www.sermo.com/resources/side-hustle-for-doctors/.
- Medical Job Board. Look for Zebras. https://lookforzebras.com/.
- Platform for Growing a Mental Health Practice. Headway. https://headway.co/for-providers#get-started
- Untapped Physician Careers. Doctoring Differently. https://www.doctoringdifferently.com/#_uuglg06xm
- Medical Expert Witness Resources SEAK. https://seak.com/.

Appendix J
Telemedicine Companies

- **98point6**
  https://www.98point6.com/
- **Access TeleCare**
  https://www.accesstelecare.com/
- **Accolade**
  https://www.accolade.com/
- **Alma**
  https://helloalma.com/
- **Amazon One Medical**
  https://onemedical.com/
- **Amwell**
  https://business.amwell.com/
- **Avel eCare**
  https://www.avelecare.com/
- **Brightside Health**
  https://www.brightside.com/
- **Care Centrix**
  https://www.carecentrix.com/
- **Change Healthcare/Optum**
  https://changehealthcare.com/
- **Charlie Health**
  https://www.charliehealth.com/
- **CirrusMD**
  https://cirrusmd.com/
- **Click Therapeutics**
  https://clicktherapeutics.com/
- **CVS Health**
  https://www.cvshealth.com/

- **DispatchHealth**
  https://www.dispatchhealth.com/
- **Doctor on Demand**
  https://doctorondemand.com/
- **Doximity**
  https://www.doximity.com/
- **GoodRx**
  https://www.goodrx.com/
- **Grow Therapy**
  https://growtherapy.com/
- **HealthJoy**
  https://healthjoy.com/
- **HealthTap**
  https://www.healthtap.com/
- **Hims & Hers Health**
  https://www.forhims.com/
  https://www.forhers.com/
- **Jabra Hearing**
  https://www.jabra.com/
- **LiveHealth Online**
  https://livehealthonline.com/
- **Maven**
  https://www.mavenclinic.com/
- **Maxim Healthcare**
  https://maximhealthcare.com/
- **MD Live**
  https://www.mdlive.com/
- **MeMD**
  https://www.memd.me/
- **Nourish**
  https://www.nourishhealth.com/
- **NuvoAir** Medical
  https://nuvoair.com/

- **Optimize Health**
  https://vivocaresolutions.com/
- **Optum Now**
  https://now.optum.com/
- **Plum**
  https://plumhealthdpc.com
- **PlushCare**
  https://www.plushcare.com/
- **Ro**
  https://ro.co/
- **Sesame Care**
  https://sesamecare.com/
- **SimplePractice**
  https://www.simplepractice.com/
- **SonderMind**
  https://www.sondermind.com/
- **Strive Health**
  https://strivehealth.com/
- **Talkspace**
  https://www.talkspace.com/
- **Tebra**
  https://www.tebra.com/
- **Teladoc Health**
  https://www.teladochealth.com/
- **The Clinic by Cleveland Clinic**
  https://my.clevelandclinic.org/
- **Virtuwell**
  https://virtuwell.com/
- **Wellframe**
  https://www.wellframe.com/
- **Zocdoc**
  https://www.zocdoc.com/

www.ingramcontent.com/pod-product-compliance
Lightning Source LLC
Chambersburg PA
CBHW071355230926
51846CB00002B/564
* 9 7 8 1 9 6 0 7 6 2 4 5 0 *